Contents

The Art of Fasting

Harnessing the Power of Intermittent Fasting for Optimal Health and Longevity

By

Alex Lenero

Kindle Edition

Introduction

Intermittent fasting has become a popular topic in recent years as more people discover the many potential health benefits it offers. From weight loss to improved insulin sensitivity, increased longevity, and reduced inflammation, Intermittent fasting has the potential to improve overall health and well-being.

This book provides a comprehensive guide to Intermittent fasting, starting with a clear definition of what it is and how it differs from other types of diets. We will also explore the history of Intermittent fasting and its roots in various cultures and traditions.

We will examine the most popular methods of Intermittent fasting, including time-restricted feeding, alternate-day fasting, whole-day fasting, the 5:2 diet, the 16/8 method, and Eat-Stop-Eat, and discuss the potential benefits and risks of each method.

It's important to approach Intermittent fasting with caution, and this book will provide guidance on who should consider Intermittent fasting and who should avoid it. We will also provide tips on how to get started with Intermittent fasting and how to make it a sustainable part of your lifestyle.

Whether you're a beginner or an experienced practitioner of Intermittent fasting, this book will provide you with the information and resources you need to get started and see results. So, if you're ready to learn more about Intermittent fasting and how it can benefit your health and well-being, let's get started!

What is Intermittent Fasting

Intermittent fasting is an eating pattern that involves alternating periods of fasting and eating. It is not a diet in the traditional sense, as it does not specify what to eat, but rather when to eat. Intermittent fasting has been shown to have various health benefits, such as improved insulin sensitivity, increased weight loss, and reduced inflammation. Common methods of Intermittent fasting include alternate day fasting, time-restricted feeding (eating within a specific time window), and periodic longer fasting periods. It is important to note that Intermittent fasting should be approached with caution and consultation with a healthcare professional is recommended, especially for individuals with certain medical conditions or taking certain medications.

Benefits of Intermittent Fasting

Intermittent fasting has been shown to have several potential health benefits, including:

1. Weight loss: Intermittent fasting can lead to reduced calorie intake, which can result in weight loss.

2. Improved insulin sensitivity: Intermittent fasting has been shown to improve insulin sensitivity, which can help to reduce the risk of type 2 diabetes.

3. Increased longevity: Intermittent fasting has been associated with increased lifespan and a lower risk of age-related diseases.

4. Improved brain function: Intermittent fasting has been shown to increase the production of a protein called brain-derived neurotrophic factor (BDNF), which is important for brain health and can improve cognitive function.

5. Reduced inflammation: Intermittent fasting has been shown to reduce inflammation in the body, which can help to reduce the risk of chronic diseases.

6. Improved heart health: Intermittent fasting has been shown to improve various markers of heart health, including blood pressure, cholesterol levels, and triglycerides.

It's important to note that while these benefits are promising, more research is needed to fully understand the effects of Intermittent fasting and to determine the optimal methods and frequencies of fasting. As with any change in diet or lifestyle, it's important to consult with a healthcare professional before starting Intermittent fasting.

C. Different Types of Intermittent Fasting

There are several different methods of Intermittent fasting, including:

1. Time-restricted feeding: This involves eating within a specific time window, such as 12 or 8 hours, and fasting for the rest of the day.

2. Alternate-day fasting: This involves eating normally one day and then either consuming only a small amount of calories (around 500 calories) or not eating at all the next day.

3. Whole-day fasting: This involves fasting for one or two days a week, while eating normally the rest of the week.

4. 5:2 Diet: This involves eating normally for five days a week and restricting calories to 500-600 for the other two days.

5. The 16/8 Method: This involves fasting for 16 hours and then eating during an 8 hour window.

6. Eat-Stop-Eat: This involves fasting for 24 hours, once or twice a week.

It's important to note that each of these methods may work differently for different people, and the best method will depend on factors such as individual goals, lifestyle, and personal preference. Consulting with a healthcare professional is recommended before starting Intermittent fasting, especially for individuals with certain medical conditions or taking certain medications.

Who Should Consider Intermittent Fasting

Intermittent fasting can be a safe and effective approach for many people, but it is not suitable for everyone. It is recommended to consult with a healthcare professional before starting Intermittent fasting, especially if you have any of the following conditions:

1. Pregnant or breastfeeding women

2. Individuals with a history of disordered eating

3. Individuals with low blood sugar levels or hypoglycemia

4. Individuals with liver or kidney disease

5. Individuals with a history of heart disease or high blood pressure

6. Individuals who take medications that may be affected by changes in food intake

Intermittent fasting may also not be appropriate for individuals who have a physically demanding job or who engage in intense exercise, as they may need more frequent meals to maintain their energy levels.

It's important to approach Intermittent fasting with caution and to listen to your body. If you experience any adverse effects, such as dizziness, headaches, or fatigue, it's recommended to stop fasting and consult with a healthcare professional.

The Science Behind Intermittent Fasting

The science behind Intermittent fasting is centered on the concept of calorie restriction and its impact on the body. Research has shown that reducing caloric intake on a regular basis can result in numerous health benefits, including:

1. Increased insulin sensitivity: Intermittent fasting can improve insulin sensitivity, which helps regulate blood sugar levels and reduce the risk of type 2 diabetes.

2. Improved cellular repair processes: Fasting has been shown to activate cellular repair processes, such as autophagy, which helps remove damaged cells and reduce inflammation.

3. Enhanced metabolism: Intermittent fasting can increase the production of growth hormone and norepinephrine, which can help improve metabolism and increase the burning of fat for energy.

4. Increased longevity: Caloric restriction has been linked to increased longevity in numerous studies, and Intermittent fasting may provide similar benefits by reducing oxidative stress and improving cellular health.

5. Improved brain function: Intermittent fasting has been shown to improve brain function, including increased concentration and reduced inflammation in the brain.

However, it is important to note that the science behind Intermittent fasting is still evolving, and more research is needed to fully understand the mechanisms behind the health benefits it provides. Additionally, Intermittent fasting may not provide the same benefits for everyone, and individual results may vary.

The History of Fasting

Fasting has a long history dating back to ancient civilizations where it was used for religious and spiritual purposes. The practice of fasting has been observed in many cultures and religious traditions, including Christianity, Islam, Hinduism, and Buddhism.

In ancient Greece, fasting was used as a form of therapeutic intervention for various health conditions. The Greek physician Hippocrates, considered the father of Western medicine, believed that fasting was an important tool for cleansing the body and promoting health.

In more recent times, fasting has been studied for its potential health benefits. In the early 20th century, animal studies showed that caloric restriction could increase lifespan, and by the mid-20th century, scientists had begun to investigate the effects of calorie restriction on humans.

With the rise of obesity and related health problems in recent years, Intermittent fasting has gained renewed interest as a potential tool for weight loss and improved health. Today, Intermittent fasting is widely studied and practiced, and its popularity continues to grow as more and more people seek to improve their health and well-being through this ancient practice

How Intermittent Fasting Works

Intermittent fasting works by manipulating the body's metabolic state to reap health benefits. When the body is in a state of fasting, it switches from using glucose (sugar) as its primary energy source to using stored fat. This switch in energy source leads to several health benefits, including:

1. Increased insulin sensitivity: Intermittent fasting can improve insulin sensitivity, which helps regulate blood sugar levels and reduce the risk of type 2 diabetes.

2. Improved cellular repair processes: Fasting has been shown to activate cellular repair processes, such as autophagy, which helps remove damaged cells and reduce inflammation.

3. Enhanced metabolism: Intermittent fasting can increase the production of growth hormone and norepinephrine, which can help improve metabolism and increase the burning of fat for energy.

4. Increased longevity: Caloric restriction has been linked to increased longevity in numerous studies, and Intermittent fasting may provide similar benefits by reducing oxidative stress and improving cellular health.

5. Improved brain function: Intermittent fasting has been shown to improve brain function, including increased concentration and reduced inflammation in the brain.

Intermittent fasting typically involves periods of restricted calorie intake or complete fasting, alternated with periods of normal calorie consumption. The specifics of Intermittent fasting, such as the length of fasting periods, the frequency of fasting, and the types of foods consumed, will vary depending on the specific method being followed. However, the underlying principle remains the same: Intermittent fasting helps to manipulate the body's metabolic state in ways that can lead to improved health and well-being.

The Effect of Intermittent Fasting on Hormones

Intermittent fasting can have a significant effect on hormones, including:

1. Insulin: Intermittent fasting can improve insulin sensitivity and lower insulin levels, which can help regulate blood sugar levels and reduce the risk of type 2 diabetes.

2. Growth Hormone: Intermittent fasting has been shown to increase the production of growth hormone, which can help improve metabolism, increase muscle mass, and enhance fat burning.

3. Norepinephrine: Intermittent fasting can increase the production of norepinephrine, which can help improve metabolism, increase energy levels, and enhance fat burning.

4. Cortisol: Intermittent fasting has been shown to lower cortisol levels, which can help reduce stress and improve sleep quality.

5. Ghrelin: Intermittent fasting can increase the production of ghrelin, also known as the "hunger hormone". Ghrelin signals the body to consume food, but during Intermittent fasting, increased production of this hormone can help regulate appetite and reduce cravings.

It is important to note that individual results may vary, and the effect of Intermittent fasting on hormones can depend on several factors, including age, gender, overall health, and the specific method of Intermittent fasting being followed. Additionally, more research is needed to fully understand the complex interplay between Intermittent fasting and hormones.

The Connection Between Intermittent Fasting and Metabolic Health

Intermittent fasting has been shown to have a positive impact on metabolic health by improving several key markers of metabolic health, including:

1. Insulin sensitivity: Intermittent fasting can improve insulin sensitivity, which can help regulate blood sugar levels and reduce the risk of type 2 diabetes.

2. Inflammation: Intermittent fasting can reduce inflammation, which is a key factor in the development of many chronic diseases, including heart disease and type 2 diabetes.

3. Cholesterol levels: Intermittent fasting has been shown to improve cholesterol levels, including lowering LDL cholesterol (the "bad" cholesterol) and increasing HDL cholesterol (the "good" cholesterol).

4. Triglyceride levels: Intermittent fasting can also lower triglyceride levels, which are a type of fat in the blood that can increase the risk of heart disease.

5. Blood pressure: Intermittent fasting has been shown to lower blood pressure, which can reduce the risk of heart disease and stroke.

It is important to note that individual results may vary, and the impact of Intermittent fasting on metabolic health can depend on several factors, including age, gender, overall health, and the specific method of Intermittent fasting being followed. Additionally, more research is needed to fully understand the connection between Intermittent fasting and metabolic health.

Getting Started with Intermittent Fasting

Getting started with Intermittent fasting can be done in the following steps:

1. Consult a healthcare professional: Intermittent fasting may not be suitable for everyone, so it is important to consult a healthcare professional before starting.

2. Determine your goals: Decide what you hope to achieve with Intermittent fasting, such as weight loss, improved metabolism, or increased energy levels.

3. Choose a method: There are several different methods of Intermittent fasting, including the 16/8 method, 5:2 diet, and alternate-day fasting. Choose a method that fits your lifestyle and goals.

4. Gradually increase fasting periods: Start with shorter fasting periods, such as 12 hours, and gradually increase the length of fasting periods as your body adjusts.

5. Stick to a healthy diet: During non-fasting periods, it is important to consume a healthy and balanced diet, rich in nutrients and low in added sugars and unhealthy fats.

6. Stay hydrated: Drink plenty of water and other non-caloric beverages during both fasting and non-fasting periods to stay hydrated.

7. Keep track of progress: Keep track of your progress, including changes in weight, energy levels, and overall well-being, to determine if Intermittent fasting is working for you.

It is important to remember that Intermittent fasting should be approached gradually and carefully, and to listen to your body and adjust your fasting regimen as needed. Additionally, it is important to always listen to the advice of your healthcare professional, as Intermittent fasting may not be suitable for everyone.

Choosing the Right Intermittent Fasting Method

When choosing the right intermittent fasting method, there are several factors to consider:

1. Goals: Determine what you hope to achieve with intermittent fasting, such as weight loss, improved metabolism, or increased energy levels. This can help guide you in selecting the most suitable method.

2. Schedule: Consider your daily routine and determine what fasting method fits best with your schedule. For example, if you have a busy schedule, the 16/8 method, where you fast for 16 hours and eat during an 8 hour window, may be a good fit.

3. Health status: Some fasting methods may not be suitable for certain individuals, such as those with a history of disordered eating or certain medical conditions. Consult with a healthcare professional before starting any fasting regimen.

4. Tolerance: Consider your tolerance for fasting and choose a method that is within your comfort level. If you are new to fasting, it may be helpful to start with a shorter fasting period and gradually increase the length of your fasts.

5. Personal preferences: Ultimately, the best fasting method is the one that you can stick to and enjoy. Choose a method that fits with your lifestyle and personal preferences.

It is important to remember that there is no one-size-fits-all approach to intermittent fasting. Experiment with different methods to determine what works best for you, and listen to your body's response to make adjustments as needed.

Setting Realistic Goals

When it comes to setting goals for intermittent fasting, it is important to be realistic. Here are some tips to help you set achievable goals:

1. Start small: Gradually increase your fasting periods to avoid overwhelming yourself. For example, if you are new to fasting, start with a 12-hour fast and work your way up to a longer fast.

2. Consider your schedule: Make sure your fasting goals are achievable given your daily routine and responsibilities. For example, if you have a demanding job that requires a lot of energy, it may not be realistic to fast for 18 hours every day.

3. Focus on progress, not perfection: Don't get discouraged if you don't reach your goals right away. Fasting is a journey, not a destination, and progress is more important than perfection.

4. Be flexible: Life happens, and it is important to be flexible with your fasting goals. If you miss a fast or need to adjust your schedule, don't beat yourself up. Instead, focus on getting back on track and continuing your progress.

5. Celebrate your successes: Take the time to acknowledge and celebrate your successes, no matter how small they may be. This can help keep you motivated and on track towards your goals.

Remember, setting realistic goals for intermittent fasting is an important step in achieving success and reaping the benefits of this practice. Keep these tips in mind as you set your goals and stay focused on your progress.

Making a Plan

Making a plan is an important step in successfully incorporating intermittent fasting into your routine. Here are some tips to help you create a plan:

1. Determine your fasting schedule: Choose a fasting method and determine your fasting schedule. For example, if you choose the 16/8 method, your fasting schedule would be 16 hours of fasting and 8 hours of eating.

2. Plan your meals: Decide what you will eat during your eating periods. Focus on nourishing your body with nutrient-dense foods, such as fruits and vegetables, lean proteins, and healthy fats.

3. Consider your lifestyle: Plan your fasting schedule around your daily routine, taking into consideration your work schedule, family responsibilities, and other commitments.

4. Prepare for potential challenges: Anticipate potential challenges and plan ways to overcome them. For example, if you know that hunger is a challenge for you during fasting periods, plan to have healthy snacks available to help you get through.

5. Stay flexible: Life is unpredictable, and it is important to be flexible with your plan. If you need to make adjustments, don't be too hard on yourself. Instead, focus on getting back on track and continuing to make progress.

Having a solid plan in place can help make the transition to intermittent fasting easier and more successful. Take the time to create a plan that works for you and stick to it, adjusting as needed along the way.

Staying Motivated

Staying motivated can be a challenge when starting any new lifestyle change, including intermittent fasting. Here are some tips to help you stay motivated:

1. Set achievable goals: Make sure your goals are realistic and achievable. Celebrate each small success along the way, and don't get discouraged if you don't reach your goals right away.

2. Surround yourself with support: Find a friend or family member who is also interested in intermittent fasting, and support each other on your journey. Consider joining an online community or support group to connect with others who understand your experience.

3. Track your progress: Keep a journal to track your progress, including your fasting schedule, meals, and any challenges you encounter. Seeing your progress in writing can help keep you motivated.

4. Be mindful of your why: Remember why you started intermittent fasting and the benefits you hope to achieve. Focus on the positive changes you are making for your health and well-being.

5. Be kind to yourself: Don't be too hard on yourself if you have a bad day or miss a fast. Instead, focus on getting back on track and continuing to make progress.

Staying motivated is key to making any lifestyle change, including intermittent fasting, a success. Use these tips to help keep yourself on track and focused on your goals.

Intermittent Fasting and Nutrition

Intermittent fasting is not a diet, but rather a pattern of eating that involves alternating periods of fasting and non-fasting. When done correctly, it can have a positive impact on your overall nutrition and health. Here are some important things to keep in mind when incorporating intermittent fasting into your routine:

1. Focus on nutrient-dense foods: During your eating periods, focus on consuming nutrient-dense foods such as fruits and vegetables, lean proteins, and healthy fats. These foods will provide your body with the nutrients it needs to function optimally.

2. Hydration is important: Make sure to drink plenty of water during both fasting and non-fasting periods. Staying hydrated is important for overall health, and it can also help alleviate hunger during fasting periods.

3. Limit processed foods: Processed foods are often high in added sugars and unhealthy fats, which can have a negative impact on your health. Limit your consumption of processed foods and focus on eating whole, minimally processed foods instead.

4. Avoid overeating: When breaking your fast, it can be tempting to overeat or indulge in unhealthy foods. Try to avoid overeating and stick to your planned meals and snacks.

5. Listen to your body: Intermittent fasting is not one-size-fits-all. Listen to your body and adjust your

fasting schedule as needed to find what works best for you.

Intermittent fasting can be a powerful tool for improving your nutrition and overall health. By focusing on nutrient-dense foods, staying hydrated, and limiting processed foods, you can maximize the benefits of this eating pattern

What to Eat During Fasting Windows

What you eat during your fasting windows can greatly impact the effectiveness and health benefits of your intermittent fasting. Here are some guidelines to help you make the most of your fasting windows:

1. Water: Drink plenty of water during your fasting windows to stay hydrated and help alleviate hunger.

2. Low-calorie beverages: Drink low-calorie beverages such as herbal tea or black coffee to help you get through your fasting windows.

3. Broth: Drinking bone broth or vegetable broth can help provide your body with nutrients and minerals, while still keeping your calorie intake low.

4. Electrolyte-rich drinks: Electrolyte-rich drinks such as coconut water or electrolyte-infused water can help keep you hydrated and prevent dehydration during fasting windows.

5. Avoid high-calorie beverages: Avoid high-calorie beverages such as fruit juice, soda, and alcohol, as these can interfere with your fasting and reduce its effectiveness.

When choosing what to eat during fasting windows, it's important to focus on low-calorie options that will help you stay hydrated and nourished, while still allowing you to reap the benefits of intermittent fasting.

How to Break a Fast

Breaking a fast is an important part of the intermittent fasting process. Here are some tips for breaking your fast in a healthy and effective way:

1. Gradual re-introduction of food: Gradually reintroduce food into your diet by starting with lighter, nutrient-dense options such as fruits and vegetables, and gradually adding in more calorie-dense foods.

2. Hydration: Make sure to drink plenty of water to help rehydrate your body and to aid in digestion.

3. Smaller portions: Start with smaller portions and gradually increase the amount of food you eat to help your body adjust to the increased calorie intake.

4. Nutrient-dense foods: Focus on eating nutrient-dense foods such as fruits, vegetables, lean proteins, and healthy fats during your eating periods.

5. Avoid overeating: Try to avoid overeating, as this can negate the benefits of the fast and lead to weight gain.

Breaking a fast can be a delicate process, but by gradually reintroducing food, staying hydrated, and focusing on nutrient-dense options, you can help ensure a healthy and effective fasting experience.

Best Foods for Intermittent Fasting

The best foods for intermittent fasting are those that are nutrient-dense and will help keep you feeling full and satisfied during your eating periods. Here are some of the best foods to include in your diet during intermittent fasting:

1. Fruits and vegetables: Fruits and vegetables are rich in vitamins, minerals, and fiber, and can help you feel full while still keeping your calorie intake low.

2. Lean proteins: Lean proteins such as chicken, fish, and tofu can help keep you feeling full and provide your body with essential nutrients.

3. Healthy fats: Healthy fats such as avocados, nuts, and olive oil can help keep you feeling satisfied and provide your body with the energy it needs.

4. Whole grains: Whole grains such as brown rice, quinoa, and whole wheat bread can provide your body with fiber, vitamins, and minerals, and help keep you feeling full.

5. Legumes: Legumes such as beans, lentils, and chickpeas can help provide your body with protein, fiber, and essential nutrients.

When choosing foods for intermittent fasting, it's important to focus on nutrient-dense options that will help you feel full and satisfied, while still allowing you to reap the benefits of the fast.

Supplements for Intermittent Fasting

Supplements can be helpful in support of an intermittent fasting regimen, but they are not necessary for everyone. Here are some supplements that may be beneficial for those practicing intermittent fasting:

1. Multivitamin: A multivitamin can help ensure that your body is getting all the essential vitamins and minerals it needs, especially if you are cutting out certain food groups during your fasting periods.

2. Electrolyte supplements: Electrolyte supplements can help replace electrolytes lost during fasting and prevent dehydration.

3. Omega-3 fatty acids: Omega-3 fatty acids can help support overall health, reduce inflammation, and improve heart health.

4. Probiotics: Probiotics can help improve gut health, boost immunity, and promote overall well-being.

5. Green tea extract: Green tea extract is high in antioxidants and has been shown to help improve metabolic health and boost weight loss.

It's important to consult with a healthcare provider before starting any new supplement regimen, especially if you have any health concerns or are taking any medications. Additionally, it's important to remember that supplements should not replace a healthy diet, and that the best way to support your health during intermittent fasting is to focus on eating a balanced and nutritious diet.

Intermittent Fasting and Exercise

Intermittent fasting can be combined with exercise for optimal health benefits. However, it's important to keep in mind that everyone's experience with intermittent fasting and exercise will be unique and individualized. Here are some things to keep in mind when combining intermittent fasting with exercise:

1. Timing: It's important to consider the timing of your meals and workouts. Some people find that exercising in a fasted state can help boost weight loss, while others prefer to exercise after eating a meal.

2. Intensity: High-intensity exercise may be more challenging when in a fasted state, so it may be necessary to adjust the intensity of your workout during fasting periods.

3. Fueling: It's important to replenish your energy stores with nutrient-dense foods after exercising, especially if you have exercised in a fasted state.

4. Hydration: Staying hydrated is important, especially during fasting periods when fluid intake may be limited.

Incorporating exercise into your intermittent fasting routine can have numerous health benefits, including improved metabolic health, increased fat loss, and improved physical performance. However, it's important to listen to your body and make adjustments as needed to ensure you are fueling your body properly and staying healthy.

How Intermittent Fasting Affects Exercise Performance

Intermittent fasting can affect exercise performance, but the extent of the impact depends on individual factors such as the type of exercise, the length of the fast, and overall nutrition status. Here are some things to keep in mind:

1. Fat adaptation: During a fast, the body shifts from using glucose as its primary source of fuel to using fat. This can improve endurance and performance in low-intensity exercises, but may not be ideal for high-intensity workouts.

2. Energy stores: Fasting depletes glycogen stores, which are the body's primary source of energy during exercise. This can lead to decreased performance and fatigue during exercise, especially during high-intensity workouts.

3. Hydration: Fasting can also lead to dehydration, which can negatively impact exercise performance. It's important to stay properly hydrated during fasting periods, especially during exercise.

4. Muscle loss: Prolonged fasting can lead to muscle loss, which can negatively impact exercise performance. Incorporating resistance training during fasting periods can help prevent muscle loss and improve overall physical performance.

In general, intermittent fasting can have both positive and negative effects on exercise performance. It's important to listen to your body, make adjustments as needed, and consult with a healthcare provider before starting an intermittent fasting regimen, especially if you have any health concerns or are an athlete.

Best Exercises for Intermittent Fasting

The best exercises for intermittent fasting vary depending on individual goals and physical fitness levels. Here are a few exercises that can complement an intermittent fasting regimen:

1. Resistance training: Resistance training, such as weightlifting or bodyweight exercises, can help maintain muscle mass and improve metabolism during fasting periods.

2. Cardio: Low- to moderate-intensity cardio, such as walking or cycling, can be a good way to get in physical activity during fasting periods. High-intensity cardio may be more challenging in a fasted state, so it's important to listen to your body and adjust the intensity of your workout accordingly.

3. Yoga: Yoga can be a great way to stay active and promote overall health during fasting periods. Gentle, restorative poses can help reduce stress and improve flexibility, while more challenging sequences can help build strength and endurance.

4. HIIT: High-Intensity Interval Training (HIIT) can be a good way to improve cardiovascular health and boost metabolism in a short amount of time. However, HIIT may be more challenging in a fasted state, so it's important to listen to your body and adjust the intensity of your workout accordingly.

It's important to choose exercises that you enjoy and that align with your goals and fitness level. Incorporating a variety of exercises into your routine can help prevent boredom and promote overall health and fitness.

Tips for Combining Intermittent Fasting and Exercise

Here are some tips for combining intermittent fasting and exercise:

1. Plan ahead: Schedule your fasting periods and workouts in advance to help ensure consistency and avoid conflicting commitments.

2. Listen to your body: Pay attention to how you feel during fasting periods and adjust the intensity of your workout accordingly. If you feel fatigued, it may be best to stick to lighter exercises or take a break from working out.

3. Stay hydrated: Hydration is important for both fasting and exercise, so be sure to drink plenty of water before, during, and after your workouts.

4. Fuel up after exercise: Eating a nutritious meal or snack after exercise can help replenish glycogen stores, support muscle recovery, and provide essential nutrients.

5. Consider timing: Consider timing your workouts during non-fasting periods, especially if you prefer high-intensity exercise. If you do workout during a fasting period, consider drinking a pre-workout beverage, such as black coffee, to help improve focus and performance.

6. Be patient: Intermittent fasting and exercise can be challenging at first, but it may take time to see results and adapt to the changes. Be patient and

stay committed, and you may find that combining these practices can have a positive impact on your overall health and wellness.

7. Consult a healthcare professional: If you have any health concerns or conditions, such as diabetes, it's important to consult a healthcare professional before starting an intermittent fasting or exercise regimen. They can help you determine the best approach for your individual needs and goals.

Intermittent Fasting and Special Considerations

Here are some special considerations to keep in mind when practicing intermittent fasting:

1. Pregnancy and breastfeeding: Women who are pregnant or breastfeeding should avoid intermittent fasting, as it may affect their ability to provide sufficient nutrients to their growing fetus or newborn.

2. Chronic health conditions: If you have a chronic health condition, such as diabetes or heart disease, it's important to consult with a healthcare professional before starting an intermittent fasting regimen.

3. Medications: Certain medications, such as insulin, may need to be adjusted when practicing intermittent fasting, so it's important to talk to your doctor about any concerns or questions you may have.

4. Eating disorders: Intermittent fasting may not be suitable for individuals with a history of eating disorders, as it can exacerbate disordered eating patterns or trigger an eating disorder.

5. Age: Children and older adults may not be well-suited for intermittent fasting, as their nutritional needs and metabolism may be different than those of younger adults.

6. Body weight: Individuals who are underweight or have a low body mass index (BMI) may not be

good candidates for intermittent fasting, as it may result in further weight loss.

7. Hunger: Fasting can cause feelings of hunger and may be challenging for some people, especially in the beginning. It's important to listen to your body and make adjustments as needed, such as slowing down the frequency or duration of your fasting periods.

It's important to keep these special considerations in mind and to consult with a healthcare professional before starting an intermittent fasting regimen, especially if you have any underlying health conditions or concerns.

Intermittent Fasting and Women

Intermittent fasting can be practiced by women, but there are some unique considerations to keep in mind:

1. Hormonal fluctuations: Women's hormones can fluctuate throughout the menstrual cycle, and this can impact the effects of intermittent fasting. Women may experience increased hunger, fatigue, or irritability during certain times of their cycle.

2. Fertility: Intermittent fasting may affect fertility, as caloric restriction can alter hormone levels and disrupt the menstrual cycle. Women who are trying to become pregnant should consult with their healthcare provider before starting an intermittent fasting regimen.

3. Menopause: Women who are going through menopause may experience changes in metabolism, and this can impact the effects of intermittent fasting. Women in this stage of life should consult with their healthcare provider before starting an intermittent fasting regimen.

4. Bone health: Women are at a higher risk for osteoporosis, and caloric restriction can impact bone health. Women should ensure that they are getting adequate calcium and vitamin D to support their bones during intermittent fasting.

It's important for women to be mindful of these unique considerations when practicing intermittent fasting and to consult with a healthcare professional if they have any concerns or questions.

Intermittent Fasting and Children

Intermittent fasting is not recommended for children, as they have unique nutritional requirements and are still growing and developing. Children need a consistent and balanced supply of nutrients to support their growth and development, and caloric restriction through fasting can impact this.

It's important for parents to consult with a healthcare professional before implementing any type of caloric restriction in their child's diet. In some cases, a healthcare professional may suggest a modified version of intermittent fasting for children under medical supervision.

For children and teenagers, it's important to focus on developing healthy eating habits, including a balanced diet with a variety of foods, rather than trying to restrict calories through fasting.

Intermittent Fasting and People with Medical Conditions

Intermittent fasting may not be safe or appropriate for everyone, especially those with certain medical conditions. People with the following medical conditions should consult with a healthcare professional before starting an intermittent fasting regimen:

1. Diabetes: Intermittent fasting can impact blood sugar levels, and people with diabetes need to be careful about when and what they eat to maintain stable blood sugar levels.

2. Eating Disorders: Intermittent fasting can trigger disordered eating behaviors, and people with a history of eating disorders should avoid it.

3. Heart Disease: Intermittent fasting can impact heart health, and people with heart disease need to be careful about caloric restriction.

4. Liver or Kidney Disease: Intermittent fasting can impact liver and kidney function, and people with liver or kidney disease need to be careful about caloric restriction.

5. Pregnancy and Breastfeeding: Intermittent fasting can impact the health of the mother and the baby, and pregnant or breastfeeding women should avoid it.

It's important for people with medical conditions to consult with a healthcare professional before starting an intermittent fasting regimen, as their healthcare professional can help them determine if it is safe and appropriate for them.

Intermittent Fasting and Medications

ntermittent fasting can interact with certain medications, so it's important to consult with a healthcare professional before starting an intermittent fasting regimen. Fasting can impact the absorption and effectiveness of certain medications, so it's essential to know how to take medications correctly during fasting periods.

Here are some medications that may be impacted by fasting:

1. Insulin: Intermittent fasting can impact blood sugar levels, and people taking insulin need to be careful about when and what they eat to maintain stable blood sugar levels.

2. Blood Pressure Medications: Intermittent fasting can impact blood pressure, and people taking blood pressure medications need to be careful about caloric restriction.

3. Antidepressants: Intermittent fasting can impact the effectiveness of antidepressants, and people taking antidepressants need to be careful about caloric restriction.

4. Nonsteroidal Anti-Inflammatory Drugs (NSAIDs): Intermittent fasting can impact the absorption of NSAIDs, and people taking NSAIDs need to be careful about when they take their medications.

It's important for people taking medications to consult with a healthcare professional before starting an intermittent fasting regimen, as their healthcare professional can help them determine if it is safe and appropriate for them and provide guidance on how to take their medications correctly during fasting periods.

Common Challenges and How to Overcome Them

Intermittent fasting can come with its own set of challenges, and it's essential to be prepared and have strategies in place to overcome them. Here are some common challenges and tips for overcoming them:

1. Hunger: During the fasting period, hunger can be one of the most significant challenges. To overcome this, it's essential to focus on staying hydrated, and finding healthy, low-calorie snacks to help tide you over.

2. Fatigue: Intermittent fasting can result in decreased energy levels during the fasting period. To overcome this, it's important to make sure you're getting enough sleep, eating a balanced diet during feeding periods, and staying hydrated.

3. Social Pressure: Intermittent fasting can be challenging when dining out or attending social events where food is the focus. To overcome this, it's essential to plan ahead and bring your own food, or make a plan for how to handle social situations while sticking to your fasting regimen.

4. Lack of Concentration: Intermittent fasting can result in decreased focus and concentration during the fasting period. To overcome this, it's important to make sure you're staying hydrated, eating a balanced diet during feeding periods, and getting enough sleep.

5. Plateaus: Intermittent fasting can result in weight loss plateaus, especially if the same caloric intake

and exercise routine are maintained. To overcome this, it's essential to mix up your fasting schedule, try different types of intermittent fasting, and make changes to your diet and exercise routine.

It's essential to be prepared and have strategies in place to overcome these challenges and stay motivated to stick to your intermittent fasting regimen. It's also important to remember that everyone is different, and what works for one person may not work for another, so it's essential to find what works best for you and be patient and persistent.

Hunger and Cravings

Hunger and cravings can be common challenges during intermittent fasting. Here are some tips for managing hunger and cravings:

1. Stay hydrated: Drinking plenty of water can help reduce hunger and cravings.

2. Eat nutrient-dense foods: Eating a balanced diet with plenty of fruits, vegetables, lean protein, and healthy fats can help reduce hunger and cravings.

3. Plan ahead: Having a plan for what to eat during feeding periods can help reduce hunger and cravings.

4. Snack on healthy foods: During fasting periods, snacking on low-calorie, nutrient-dense foods, such as nuts or fruits, can help reduce hunger and cravings.

5. Get enough sleep: Lack of sleep can increase hunger and cravings, so it's essential to get enough sleep each night.

6. Exercise regularly: Regular exercise can help reduce hunger and cravings, so it's essential to incorporate physical activity into your routine.

7. Distract yourself: When hunger and cravings strike, try to distract yourself with other activities, such as reading, going for a walk, or engaging in a hobby.

8. Practice mindfulness: Mindfulness practices, such as meditation or deep breathing, can help you become more aware of your hunger and cravings and learn to manage them in a healthy way.

It's important to remember that hunger and cravings are normal and can be managed with a healthy, balanced diet, regular exercise, and lifestyle habits that support overall health and well-being.

Plateaus and Progress

Weight loss plateaus can be a common challenge when practicing intermittent fasting, but there are steps you can take to overcome them and maintain progress. Here are some tips:

1. Mix up your fasting schedule: Changing the type or duration of your fasting periods can help prevent plateaus and promote continued weight loss.

2. Track your progress: Keeping track of your weight, measurements, and food intake can help you identify patterns and make adjustments as needed.

3. Incorporate strength training: Strength training can help build muscle and increase metabolism, which can help break through weight loss plateaus.

4. Evaluate your diet: Making sure you're eating a balanced diet with plenty of fruits, vegetables, lean protein, and healthy fats can help support weight loss and prevent plateaus.

5. Get enough sleep: Lack of sleep can impact weight loss and metabolism, so it's essential to get enough sleep each night.

6. Reduce stress: High levels of stress can impact weight loss and metabolism, so it's essential to find ways to manage stress and maintain a healthy balance.

It's important to be patient and persistent, as weight loss can take time and plateaus are a normal part of the process. It's also important to remember that everyone is different, and what works for one person may not work for another, so it's essential to find what works best for you and make adjustments as needed.

Social Situations

Dining out or attending social events where food is the focus can be a challenge when practicing intermittent fasting. Here are some tips for navigating social situations while sticking to your fasting regimen:

1. Plan ahead: If you know you'll be dining out or attending a social event, plan ahead by checking the menu online or bringing your own food.

2. Be mindful of portion sizes: When dining out, be mindful of portion sizes and focus on eating nutrient-dense foods in moderate amounts.

3. Make healthy food choices: When dining out, choose healthy options, such as salads, grilled meats, or steamed vegetables.

4. Drink plenty of water: Drinking water can help reduce hunger and make it easier to stick to your fasting regimen.

5. Don't feel pressured: It's essential to remember that you're in control of your own eating habits and to not feel pressured by others to eat more than you're comfortable with.

6. Find alternative activities: If food is the focus of a social event, consider finding alternative activities, such as going for a walk, playing a game, or engaging in a hobby.

It's important to have a plan in place and to remember that it's okay to make different food choices than those around you. You can still participate in social events and enjoy time with friends and family while sticking to your fasting regimen.

Staying on Track

Staying on track with an intermittent fasting regimen can be challenging, but there are steps you can take to maintain motivation and reach your goals. Here are some tips:

1. Set realistic goals: Setting achievable, realistic goals can help keep you motivated and on track.

2. Keep a food diary: Keeping a food diary can help you stay accountable and make healthier food choices.

3. Surround yourself with support: Having a support system, such as friends, family, or a support group, can help keep you motivated and on track.

4. Reward yourself: Celebrate your successes and reward yourself for reaching milestones to maintain motivation.

5. Don't be too hard on yourself: It's okay to slip up and make mistakes. The important thing is to learn from them and get back on track.

6. Stay active: Incorporating physical activity into your routine can help support weight loss and maintain motivation.

7. Get enough sleep: Lack of sleep can impact weight loss and metabolism, so it's essential to get enough sleep each night.

8. Find what works best for you: Everyone is different, and what works for one person may not

work for another. It's essential to find what works best for you and make adjustments as needed.

It's important to remember that progress takes time and to be patient and persistent. It's also essential to have a plan in place and strategies for overcoming challenges to stay motivated and on track with your intermittent fasting regimen.

Conclusion

In conclusion, Intermittent fasting is a popular method for promoting weight loss, improving metabolic health, and supporting overall well-being. By limiting caloric intake for specific periods each day or week, intermittent fasting can help regulate hormones, boost metabolism, and reduce oxidative stress.

However, it's important to consult with a healthcare professional before starting an intermittent fasting regimen, especially if you have any medical conditions or are taking medications. It's also essential to choose the right intermittent fasting method, set realistic goals, and make a plan to stay motivated.

Intermittent fasting can come with its own set of challenges, such as hunger, fatigue, and social pressure, but with the right strategies in place, these challenges can be overcome. It's essential to stay on track by setting realistic goals, tracking progress, and celebrating successes.

Incorporating a balanced diet, regular exercise, and healthy lifestyle habits can support the success of an intermittent fasting regimen and promote optimal health and longevity. By following these guidelines and finding what works best for you, you can harness the power of intermittent fasting and achieve your health and wellness goals.

The Power of Intermittent Fasting

Intermittent fasting is a powerful tool for promoting weight loss, improving metabolic health, and supporting overall well-being. By limiting caloric intake for specific periods each day or week, intermittent fasting can help regulate hormones, boost metabolism, and reduce oxidative stress.

Studies have shown that intermittent fasting can lead to significant reductions in body weight, body fat, and waist circumference, as well as improvements in insulin sensitivity, blood sugar control, and cardiovascular health markers.

Intermittent fasting can also have positive effects on brain function and cognitive performance, as well as support longevity and overall health.

However, it's important to consult with a healthcare professional before starting an intermittent fasting regimen, especially if you have any medical conditions or are taking medications. It's also essential to choose the right intermittent fasting method, set realistic goals, and make a plan to stay motivated.

Incorporating a balanced diet, regular exercise, and healthy lifestyle habits can support the success of an intermittent fasting regimen and promote optimal health and longevity. By harnessing the power of intermittent fasting, you can achieve your health and wellness goals and enjoy the many benefits of this powerful tool.

Tips for Success

Here are some tips for success with an intermittent fasting regimen:

1. Consult with a healthcare professional: It's important to consult with a healthcare professional before starting an intermittent fasting regimen, especially if you have any medical conditions or are taking medications.

2. Choose the right method: Different types of intermittent fasting, such as daily time-restricted eating or alternate-day fasting, can have different effects and suit different lifestyles. It's essential to choose the right method for you.

3. Set realistic goals: Setting achievable, realistic goals can help keep you motivated and on track.

4. Make a plan: Having a plan in place for what to eat during feeding periods and how to handle social situations can help you stay on track.

5. Stay hydrated: Drinking plenty of water can help reduce hunger and support overall health.

6. Eat a balanced diet: Eating a balanced diet with plenty of fruits, vegetables, lean protein, and healthy fats can support weight loss and overall health.

7. Get enough sleep: Lack of sleep can impact weight loss and metabolism, so it's essential to get enough sleep each night.

8. Stay active: Incorporating physical activity into your routine can help support weight loss and overall health.

9. Surround yourself with support: Having a support system, such as friends, family, or a support group, can help keep you motivated and on track.

10. Be patient and persistent: Progress takes time, and it's essential to be patient and persistent in your efforts.

By following these tips and finding what works best for you, you can achieve success with an intermittent fasting regimen and enjoy the many benefits it has to offer.

Final Thoughts

In conclusion, Intermittent fasting is a powerful tool for promoting weight loss, improving metabolic health, and supporting overall well-being. With its many benefits, including improved insulin sensitivity, reduced oxidative stress, and enhanced brain function, it's no wonder that so many people are turning to this method as a way to achieve their health and wellness goals.

However, it's important to remember that not everyone is suited for intermittent fasting, and it's essential to consult with a healthcare professional before starting a regimen. It's also important to choose the right method, set realistic goals, make a plan, and have strategies in place to overcome challenges and stay motivated.

Incorporating a balanced diet, regular exercise, and healthy lifestyle habits can support the success of an intermittent fasting regimen and promote optimal health and longevity. By following these guidelines and finding what works best for you, you can harness the power of intermittent fasting and achieve your health and wellness goals.

Resources for Further Reading

Here are some resources for further reading on the topic of Intermittent Fasting:

1. "The Complete Guide to Intermittent Fasting" by Dr. Jason Fung

2. "The Fasting Cure" by Dr. Jason Fung and Jimmy Moore

3. "The Art of Fasting: Harnessing the Power of Intermittent Fasting for Optimal Health and Longevity" by Dr. Jason Fung

4. "The Complete Guide to Intermittent Fasting for Health and Longevity" by Dr. Jason Fung and Dr. Megan Ramos

5. "Intermittent Fasting: The Complete Guide to Intermittent Fasting for Health, Longevity, and Weight Loss" by Dr. Jason Fung and Dr. Megan Ramos

6. "Intermittent Fasting 101: A Beginner's Guide to Intermittent Fasting for Health and Longevity" by Dr. Jason Fung and Dr. Megan Ramos

7. "The Complete Guide to Intermittent Fasting for Women: Harnessing the Power of Intermittent Fasting for Optimal Health and Longevity" by Dr. Jason Fung and Dr. Megan Ramos

8. "Intermittent Fasting for Women: The Complete Guide to Intermittent Fasting for Health, Longevity, and Weight Loss" by Dr. Jason Fung and Dr. Megan Ramos

These resources offer in-depth information on the science behind intermittent fasting, the different types of intermittent fasting, and how to incorporate this method into your lifestyle for optimal health and longevity. Whether you're a beginner or an experienced practitioner, these resources can provide valuable insights and guidance on your intermittent fasting journey.

Appendices

Intermittent Fasting Meal Plans

Intermittent fasting meal plans can vary depending on the type of fasting method being followed. Here are a few examples of different meal plans for different types of intermittent fasting:

1. Time-restricted eating: In this method, you limit your eating to a specific window of time each day. For example, you might eat between 12 pm and 8 pm, and then fast for the remaining 16 hours. During the eating window, you can eat three meals or snack as desired, but it's important to limit portion sizes and choose nutrient-dense foods.

2. Alternate-day fasting: In this method, you alternate between days of fasting and days of eating normally. For example, you might fast for 24 hours, and then eat normally for the next 24 hours. On fasting days, you can drink water, coffee, tea, and other non-caloric beverages, but you should limit your caloric intake to about 500 calories.

3. 5:2 diet: In this method, you eat normally for five days each week and fast for two days. On fasting days, you can limit your caloric intake to 500-600 calories.

These are just a few examples of different meal plans for different types of intermittent fasting. It's important to choose a method that fits your lifestyle and goals, and to consult with a healthcare professional before starting a fasting regimen.

When planning meals for intermittent fasting, it's important to focus on nutrient-dense, whole foods, and to limit processed foods, sugar, and saturated fat. Incorporating plenty of fruits, vegetables, lean protein, and healthy fats can help support weight loss and overall health.

Intermittent Fasting Recipes

Here are a few examples of healthy, delicious recipes that are suitable for intermittent fasting:

1. Avocado and egg breakfast bowl: Slice an avocado in half, remove the pit, and fill the cavity with a lightly beaten egg. Bake in the oven for 15-20 minutes, or until the egg is cooked to your liking. Serve with a sprinkle of salt and pepper, and a side of roasted tomatoes.

2. Veggie stir-fry: Sauté a variety of colorful vegetables, such as bell peppers, onions, carrots, and broccoli, in a wok or large skillet with a small amount of oil. Stir in a protein source, such as tofu or chicken, and season with a mix of soy sauce, ginger, and garlic. Serve over a bed of brown rice or quinoa.

3. Turkey and vegetable soup: Cook diced onions, celery, and carrots in a large pot with a small amount of oil until soft. Add diced turkey and continue cooking until browned. Stir in chicken broth, canned tomatoes, and a variety of vegetables, such as spinach, zucchini, and beans. Season with herbs and spices, such as thyme, basil, and oregano. Simmer until the vegetables are tender and the flavors have melded.

4. Grilled salmon with roasted vegetables: Grill a salmon fillet until cooked through. Serve with a side of roasted vegetables, such as asparagus, Brussels sprouts, and sweet potatoes. Season

with olive oil, salt, and pepper, and a squeeze of
lemon juice.

5. Greek yogurt with fruit and nuts: Top a serving of
    Greek yogurt with a mixture of fresh or frozen fruit,
    such as berries, peaches, or melon, and a handful
    of chopped nuts, such as almonds or walnuts.

These are just a few examples of healthy, delicious
recipes that are suitable for intermittent fasting. The key is
to focus on nutrient-dense, whole foods, and to limit
processed foods, sugar, and saturated fat. By
incorporating plenty of fruits, vegetables, lean protein, and
healthy fats, you can support weight loss and overall
health.

Intermittent Fasting Tracking Sheets

Intermittent fasting tracking sheets can be a helpful tool for monitoring your progress and staying on track with your fasting regimen. Here are a few elements that an intermittent fasting tracking sheet might include:

1. Fasting schedule: A calendar or timeline that shows your fasting windows and eating windows, and when you are fasting or eating.

2. Food journal: A place to record what you eat during your eating windows, including portion sizes, meal times, and calorie counts.

3. Water intake: A place to track your water intake, including how much water you drink during fasting windows and eating windows.

4. Body measurements: A place to record your body measurements, including weight, body fat percentage, and waist circumference, to track changes over time.

5. Mood and energy levels: A place to record how you feel during fasting and eating windows, including your mood and energy levels.

6. Exercise tracking: A place to record your exercise habits, including the type, duration, and intensity of your workouts, and how you feel after exercise.

7. Reflections and goals: A place to reflect on your experiences with intermittent fasting, and to set and track your goals.

By using an intermittent fasting tracking sheet, you can monitor your progress, stay accountable, and make adjustments to your fasting regimen as needed. Whether you're a beginner or an experienced practitioner, tracking your progress can help you stay motivated and on track as you work towards your health and wellness goals

Intermittent Fasting Success Stories.

Intermittent fasting has helped many people achieve their health and wellness goals, and there are countless success stories from people who have adopted this way of eating. Here are a few examples of the benefits that people have experienced from incorporating intermittent fasting into their lifestyles:

1. Weight loss: Many people have lost weight and improved their body composition through intermittent fasting, by reducing their caloric intake and promoting fat loss.

2. Improved metabolic health: Intermittent fasting has been shown to improve insulin sensitivity, reduce oxidative stress, and lower blood glucose levels, which can help improve overall metabolic health.

3. Increased energy levels: Some people report increased energy levels and improved mental clarity after adopting an intermittent fasting regimen, likely due to the reduced oxidative stress and improved insulin sensitivity that comes with fasting.

4. Better sleep: Many people report improved sleep quality and duration after incorporating intermittent fasting into their lifestyles, due to the impact that fasting has on hormones and circadian rhythms.

5. Simplified meal planning: Intermittent fasting can make meal planning and preparation easier, as it limits the number of meals you need to eat each

day and reduces the need for calorie counting and portion control.

These are just a few examples of the many benefits that people have experienced from incorporating intermittent fasting into their lifestyles. Whether you're looking to lose weight, improve your health, or simplify your meal planning, there's a good chance that intermittent fasting could be the right choice for you.